NURSES
ARE NUTS

(DISCUSSING HOW NURSES HELP
OTHER HOSPITAL DISCIPLINES
WHEN THEY DON'T HAVE TO)

A. E. L.

PAGE PUBLISHING, INC.
Conneaut Lake, PA

First originally published by Page Publishing 2019

ISBN 978-1-64584-778-6 (pbk)
ISBN 978-1-64584-779-3 (digital)

Printed in the United States of America

Lots of thanks to all the nurses who work tirelessly to help patients, and I hoped that nurses will one day realize the extra work that they do for multiple other professions and will one day stop or slow down considerably.

Thank you to my family members who stood beside me while writing this book, especially my daughter, Pamela.

CONTENTS

PREFACE

Nurses have one of the most, if not the most, demanding jobs in the hospital. Us nurses take care of the sick and injured in hospitals, we offer advice and emotional support for patients and families, and we sometimes, depending on the area we work, can work up to twenty-four hours straight. We admit patients, discharge patients, and take patients' vital signs, just to name a few. If nurses decided to take the day off, hospitals would be in bad shape.

Other hospital disciplines work very hard too, but the nurse's job is twenty-four-seven. Outside of having very hard jobs, nurses are also burdened with helping others with their jobs and, in some cases, doing others' jobs entirely. It is how the system is set up. I do not say that nurses are nuts to demean nurses. I say this because the system is set up for us to be found helping doctors and the volunteers with their jobs while getting little and sometimes no help from any other disciplines with our jobs.

Nurses should demand more accountability from other disciplines to do their jobs more effectively. As far as I am concerned, nurses are the backbone of the healthcare system. Nurses need to point out things to the higher-ups in hospitals, with hopes to force changes that will make the nurses' job easier.

Doctors could not get through their day without help from the nurse. When the doctor starts his day, it is the nurse that updates him on what's going on or what to expect. There are many who do not know this, but this is the case. The workers in the radiology department could not get through their day without the nurse's help. In most cases, when the radiology tech comes to get an X-ray on a patient, it is the nurse that usually identifies the correct patient that the X-ray must be taken on. When the phlebotomist comes to draw blood from a patient, he usually asks the nurse to identify the patient that the blood must be drawn from. Now the phlebotomist can easily do this on his own if he would just check the patient's name bracelet, but phlebotomists usually will never do this on their own.

Physical therapists play an important role in the hospital. They help set up equipment for patients and walk with them. Lots of a patient's progress and how a patient is doing can be found in the chart for that patient, but it is not uncommon for the physical therapist to go to the nurse to get information on the patient. This information can consist of the patient's dietary regimen and his activity level. Nurses can be found helping health-unit coordinators (HUCs) quite a bit in hospitals.

Pharmacists play a vital role in hospitals, from making intravenous solutions to supplying patients' medications. The pharmacist depends on the nurses quite a bit to get his job done.

Respiratory therapists help patients when they are having breathing issues. It is not uncommon for the respiratory therapist to get the nurse's help with many of the things that he is carrying out.

Nurses can be found doing lots of the housekeepers' duties, from sweeping floors to cleaning up spills. Nurses routinely do lots of transporting duties that patients require.

Nurses do lots of the volunteer's duties when it comes to updating family members on what is going on with their loved ones. Nurses can also be found working on duties that should be performed by registration and duties that belong to security.

DOCTORS

Even though it is the doctor's responsibility to put in patient's orders, nurses routinely pick up the slack and do it themselves, and lots of times, with very little thanks in return. Now true, we can get a verbal order from the doctor to do it, but we sometimes will do it ourselves in order not to call the doctor, which does the doctor a favor. We oftentimes assist doctors with bedside procedures, like closed reductions of joints and inserting central lines.

We can be found going into the operating rooms to help position a patient on the operating-room table to help the anesthesiologist give blood products. When the nurse has to position a patient, she does it alone. When the nurse has to give a blood product, she gives it alone. There are times, after surgery, when nurses are left to enter verbal orders for a patient because, in some cases, the surgeon forgets to do it.

There are patients that have consultations with other doctors. Lots of times, the consulting doctor will have the nurse put in orders that the consulting doctor should put in himself. Lots of times, after surgery, a patient may need to go to critical care. In lots of instances, this must be cleared with the intensivist. An intensivist is a medical specialist in critical care medicine. The intensivist needs to know if the patient meets critical care criteria. The surgeon who wants the patient to go to critical care should talk to the intensivist, but lots of times, this responsibility falls on the nurse. There are times when the doctor will trust the nurse to talk to the intensivist even though it is the doctor's job to talk to the intensivist. It is nice that nurses are trusted by doctors in some cases, but the nurse is still doing the doctor's job in these cases. It is not uncommon for the doctor to be with the nurse overseeing a patient that is not doing well, the doctor asking for specific tests and medications for the patient that requires a doctor's order, and the nurse having to put the order in because the doctor will not do it, but the doctor is supposed to do it.

There are lots of times, after procedures, when patients need specific tests, such as labs or X-rays that are not ordered. The nurse, knowing that these tests are needed, will order them and later inform the doctor that she ordered the tests. Yet again, the nurse is doing the doctor's job. When patients are going into surgery, there are things that the surgeon and anesthesiologist must know, such as the patient's lab, CXR, and EKG results. These things are in the patient's computer records and charts, and the doctor has access to them. There have been and still are times when the nurse gets in trouble for not pointing out to the doctor that there is an irregularity in one of the areas, let's say before the patient goes to surgery. The surgeon is supposed to view this material on his own. It is not the nurse's job to do this. Lots of times, after surgery, the surgeon is supposed to go talk to the patient's family members about how the surgery went. Lots of times, the surgeon fails to do this, leaving the nurse to try to explain the surgery in the best way that he can or to page the surgeon to see if he can come talk to the family members. In both of these cases, the nurse is doing the doctor's job.

The physician assistant sometimes puts in orders for physicians. Lots of times, they are not sure of what orders to put in for medications, such as for antibiotics and pain. Lots of these times, the physician assistant will talk to get clarification and input as to what to order, and the nurse will help out with this most of the time. Nurses cover for doctors when JCAHO comes to hospitals. JCAHO is an organization made up of individuals from the private medical sector to develop and maintain standard quality in medical facilities in the United States. There are many times when doctors have made documentation errors. When this happens, JCAHO usually brings it to the nurse's attention. The problem here is that the nurse did not do the documentation. Nurses have been known to try to correct the doctor's documentation. If the documentation error was made by the doctor, it should be brought to the doctor's attention. If the nurse has made a documentation error, JCAHO will not bring the nurse's documentation error to the doctor.

When patients are going into surgery, it is required that a history and physical be written on them by the surgeon and the surgical consent be signed. There are multiple times when the H&P has not been written, and the surgical consent has not been signed, and it is usually the nurse who points out to the doctor that he must sign his consent. After a patient has surgery, the surgeon is supposed to write a progress note. A progress note is a part of the medical record where healthcare professionals record details to document a patient's clinical status. There are lots of times when these progress notes are not completed after surgery. It is usually the nurse who tells the surgeon that the progress note needs to be written. There are lots of times, before surgery, when patients need antibiotics, and in lots of cases, the surgeon forgets to order the antibiotic. It is usually the nurse who tells the surgeon that he forgot to order the antibiotic. Doctors are supposed to enter their own orders on the computer. There are times when the doctor does not know how to use the computer to put orders in. When this happens, it is usually the nurse who will put the orders in or show the doctor how to put the orders on the computer.

When the doctor starts his day, it is usually the nurse that updates him on what's going on or what to expect with certain patients throughout the day. In the post-anesthesia care unit, the anesthesiologist needs paperwork that is called care riders. It is the nurse's duty to produce these forms for the anesthesiologist. On the other hand, if a nurse needs paperwork, she must do it for herself, and the anesthesiologist will not do it for her. Lots of times, the doctors order consults on patients, and there are times when the doctor who was consulted is not taking consultations. The nurse is stuck with relaying this information to the consulting doctor. Nurses are also stuck covering for doctors that run late a lot. Be it discharging a patient from the hospital on time or starting surgery, doctors sometimes run late, and when this happens, the nurse is left to talk to the patient and their families about the doctor being late. In most cases, the nurse does not know why the doctor is late, but is left to come up with something to say to the patients and their families.

Nurses, at times, continue to be their own worst enemies when it comes to doctors. For instance, I had a situation when I pre-oped a patient, which means I was getting a patient ready for surgery. However, the patient I had ended up with a respiratory problem while he was in surgery. My head nurse reviewed my notes and told me that I did not document breath sounds on my patient. I did document breath sounds, but had I not, this had no bearing on what happened to the patient in surgery. The anesthesiologist and surgeons base what they are going to do based on the CXR results and the pulmonary doctor's findings not the nurse's findings.

Patients need intravenous lines when they are in the operating room. Most of the time, the nurses start these lines in the pre-op area. Sometimes, the patient needs lines with large intravenous lines so the patient can get blood products or extra fluids. There are times when the patient has difficult veins, making starting lines with large intravenous lines very difficult. When a patient gets stuck for an intravenous line, it is painful. When this happens, the patient, at times, will get upset with the nurse for the stick. It is not uncommon for the anesthesiologist to stick a patient to get this line after the patient is asleep in the operating room, but when the anesthesiologist insists on the nurse sticking an awoke patient with difficult veins, it makes the nurse's job that much harder.

There are lots of times when doctors look for other doctors. When this happens, they have a constant habit of asking the nurse where the doctor they are looking for is at. The nurse has no way of knowing where the doctor is. What they should do is call the doctor that they are looking for. There was a case, one time, when a patient developed an infection after hip surgery. Before certain surgeries, the nurse sometimes wipes the area that the patient is going to have surgery on with an aseptic wipe. Even if this is not done, it has no bearing on the patient being cleaned before surgery since this is done in the operating room before the surgeon cuts the patient. There was once a situation where it could not be proven if the patient got the aseptic wipe from the nurse. Infectious disease wanted to hold the nurse responsible for the patient's infection when the nurse had no bearing on this. Again, the patient is prepped and cleaned in the operating room before the surgeon cuts the patient. The doctor also scrubs before surgery, yet the nurse never points this out. Chances are, the patient not being properly cleaned in the OR or the doctor not properly washing is what caused the patient to get an infection. The sad part here is that the nurses, as well as the doctors, know that the aseptic technique or lack thereof in the operating room is what is going to determine whether or not the patient gets an infection, yet nurses will hold themselves responsible if a patient gets an infection.

When there are disasters that force doctors and nurses to stay in the hospital overnight, the doctors usually get the best rooms to stay in. Nurses are lucky if they can get a room with a bed and a shower! The nurses usually complain about this amongst themselves but never bring these concerns to the proper authorities. When nurses put in orders for doctors, the doctors are supposed to sign the orders off. When the doctors sign the orders off, they say that they gave the nurse those orders. Sometimes the doctor does not sign the orders off because they say they forgot to or because they say that the nurse got the order wrong. When this happens, the nurse could get in trouble. Now, in all fairness to the doctor, sometimes the nurse can get the order wrong. This is the problem with taking verbal orders from doctors. When the nurses take these verbal orders, they are doing the doctor a favor, but when something goes wrong, it is the nurse that gets the blame. The way to eliminate this is by the nurse not taking verbal orders from doctors. The doctors should be putting in their own orders.

In the recovery room in hospitals, the PACU nurses, who are the nurses that work in the post-anesthesia care unit, take call. When nurses come in for call, it is supposed to be for patients who need emergency surgery. Lots of times, patients that have had surgery go home. If the nurses that are scheduled to go home cannot get the patient out before they go home, the call nurses have to come in. There are lots of times when the nurse cannot get the patient home in time because the doctor forgot to write a discharge order. The call nurse should not have to come in for this. They do, however, and when this happens, they are quite upset. Nurses complain to each other about this but never take the issue to whom they should, which is administration.

There are times when a patient has admission orders to the floor. Sometimes the nurse that is supposed to receive the patient complains that there is no room for the patient or that they are too busy to receive the patient. Instead of telling the doctor this, the nurse gets mad at the nurse who is sending her the patient. Lots of times, in the preoperative area where I work, the doctor comes in and talks to the patient before surgery. Lots of times, they will tell the patient that he or she will be going to surgery soon, sometimes knowing that the patient will not soon be going to surgery. When the patient is delayed, lots of times, the patient will get mad at the nurse because he is delayed, leaving the nurse to cover for the doctor. In the preoperative surgical setting, the doctors and the anesthesiologists have to sign consents. There have been times when the doctors and anesthesiologists have signed the wrong consents. This is something that should not happen when each consent has written on it what it is for. When this happens, it is the nurse who has to get new consents drawn up so the correct signature goes on the right consent. There is a form that nurses have designed themselves in the preoperative area, where nurses have to answer how long they think the surgical procedure will be. Sometimes the surgeon himself does not know how long the procedure will be! Nurses are crazy to have such a form. Sometimes the anesthesiologist will not sign off on an order that the nurse put in that the patient needs right away. For instance, there have been lots of times when a patient coming into the recovery room had lots of nausea and was vomiting. The nurse, more than likely, would give an anti-nausea med, such as Zofran, that needs an anesthesiologist's order. If the anesthesiologist did not sign off on that order, the nurse could get into trouble for helping the patient.

When the doctor starts his day, it is the nurse that updates him on what's going on. In lots of cases, patients need antibiotics before surgery starts. In these cases, the nurse often asks the doctor what antibiotic is needed, and sometimes the surgeon will wait until the patient goes into the operating room before telling the nurse what antibiotic is needed. This makes it harder on the nurse, who now has to gown up and bring the antibiotic to the room. This all could have been avoided if the doctor had just told the nurse the antibiotic that was needed before the patient went to the operating room. Sometimes the doctor will attempt to put in his orders on the computer. There have been plenty of times when the nurse has told the doctor, "I know you are busy, so I will put the order in for you." There was a time when I was in the pre-op area, getting a patient ready for surgery, and an OR nurse came to me and told me that the surgeon's history and physical that he wrote on a patient was not correct. This is something she should have told the surgeon, not me. It is the surgeon that wrote the history and physical of the patient, not me. As a nurse, I cannot do that.

It is routine for the anesthesiologist to put in pain medication and anti-nausea medication for the patient after he comes out from surgery. Sometimes, the anesthesiologist will tell the nurse to call him if the patient has any nausea or pain and that he will put the orders in. This forces the nurse to call him and try to do the best that he can to soothe the patient until he gets orders. The orders should have gone in automatically, and the anesthesiologist knows this. Sometimes the nurse, who is going to be with the patient in the operating room, will get mad at the nurse who is getting the patient ready if that nurse does not know what antibiotic the patient needs in surgery instead of bringing her concerns to the surgeon, who is the only one who knows what antibiotic the patient will need in surgery.

When a patient goes in for surgery, doctors routinely mark the spots that they are going to do surgery on. Sometimes the doctor forgets to do it, and when they do, the nurse will sometimes tell the doctor that he forgot to mark the patient. This is not the nurse's responsibility. The anesthesiologist will sometimes give the patient a nerve block, which serves to lessen the patient's pain after surgery. This is usually done just before the patient goes to surgery. Sometimes the surgeon will call the nurse to ask her or him what is taking the patient so long to go to the operating room when he knows that the anesthesiologist is performing the block. He knows that he should be asking the anesthesiologist what is taking so long.

Sometimes patients that are going to surgery come from the intensive care unit. Sometimes a patient may not have an arterial or central line, which are lines that are inserted by a doctor. Lots of times, the anesthesiologist will ask the nurse why the patient does not have these lines. This is a question that should be asked of the intensive care doctor and not the nurse.

Before patients go into surgery, they sign a surgical consent, which is a consent that contains the name of the surgeon who is going to do the procedure. The procedure has the name of the doctor who is doing the procedure on the consent. Sometimes other doctors who are going to do a procedure on the patient will add the procedure they are going to do on the same consent. This is wrong. Each surgeon must have their own consent. When this happens, the nurse must call the doctor who added his name to the first consent to tell him that he must have his own consent. This puts what the surgeon should already know on the nurse to be straightened out. The doctor is supposed to sit down and look up lab results of his patients. Sometimes the nurse will do it for him. Sometimes patients have a DNR order, which means "do not resuscitate," which simply means to let the patient die if he or she is dying. When patients are in the operating room, the DNR order cannot be followed, which means that if a patient is dying in the operating room, the anesthesiologist will have to do everything that he can to keep the patient living. There are times when the patient and his family members are not aware of this and have to be told this. There have been countless times when the nurse has told the patient and family members this when it should have been told to them by the anesthesiologist.

Sometimes residents are supposed to put in orders on patients. Residents are doctors that are training in the hospital. There are times when the resident is not aware that he has to put in orders. When this happens, the nurse usually searches for the resident to let him know that he has orders to put in, but the doctor who is overseeing the resident is the one who should notify the resident of this. There are times when a patient is going for surgery when a proxy has signed the patient's surgical consent. Sometimes the operating nurse wants more information on who the proxy is. The doctor who is operating on the patient and who could not perform the patient's surgery without a consent never concerns himself with this. If the consent is not properly signed, then the doctor can get in trouble. If he is not worried about the proxy, then the nurse shouldn't be.

When patients come from the outside for surgery, they should have a printed history and physical in their chart. If not, the doctor should have it with him. When it is not in the chart and the doctor does not have it with him, the nurse must call the doctor's office to get the history and physical faxed to the hospital so that the nurse can put this material in the patient's chart. This takes up valuable time, and the nurse could be doing other things. The nurse anesthetist works directly with the anesthesiologist in the operating room. In some hospitals, the nurse anesthetist is not allowed to put in post-operative pain medication and post-operative anti-nausea medication. When they cannot put in these orders, it falls on the nurse to do it, which puts extra work on the nurse. It's crazy that the nurse anesthetist who administers anesthesia cannot put in the patient's post-op medication orders.

When patients are scheduled for surgery, sometimes the doctor will change the surgery time, and when this happens, it should be the doctor's office that calls the patient to tell him or her of the change in surgery time. However, sometimes the nurses are told by the doctors to tell the patient about their change in surgery time. Sometimes the nurse anesthetist will administer anesthesia to the patient who is having surgery. The nurse anesthetist works under the anesthesiologist. Sometimes the anesthesiologist will like for the nurse anesthetist to see the patient he worked on before the patient goes home or is transferred to the floor. Instead of telling the nurse anesthetist this himself, the anesthesiologist will tell the nurse to tell the nurse anesthetist this when this is not the nurse's job to do.

When patients go to surgery, there are lots of times when the surgeon orders an antibiotic to be given to the patient. There are times when the patient has an allergy to the antibiotic that was ordered, and it is the nurse who always catches this error. If the error is not caught, sometimes the nurse manager will reprimand the nurse who did not alert the surgeon of his error. This is wrong because this is something that the surgeon should have known himself. Press Ganey is a group that measures patient satisfaction in the hospital. When patients are in the preoperative area, their biggest complaint is usually their concerns about what is taking so long for them to go to surgery. Press Ganey's response to this is that the nurses have to try to clear this up! How can the nurses clear this up when it is the surgeons who control what time the patient is going to go to the operating room? When doctors order labs, it is their responsibility to check the lab results, yet they will sometimes get upset with the nurse if the nurse does not bring the lab results.

There are lots of times before a patient goes into surgery when the anesthesiologist will order pre-op meds on the patient to be medicated. When the nurse gives these medications, she has to sign the medications out, but when the anesthesiologist gives these medications, he does not have to sign them out. There are times when the anesthesiologist will give these medications without telling the nurse, and when this happens, the nurse does not know that the patient was given this medication and gives the medication herself. Now if the patient has been given the medication twice, the patient can sometimes have an adverse effect, especially if narcotics were given again. If the patient has an adverse effect, it is the nurse who must treat the patient. Sometimes the anesthesiologist will come and tell the nurse that he already medicated the patient, but he should have told the nurse right after he gave the patient the medication that he medicated the patient. Had that happened, the extra work of trying to help the patient who was medicated twice would not have fallen on the nurse. Nurses do not get paid extra to be a doctor. Nurses are nuts for letting these things happen.

RADIOLOGY DEPARTMENT

The radiologist routinely takes various X-rays on patients. Lots of times, regardless of how busy the nurses are, we are expected to help the radiology tech position the patient so that the X-ray can be performed. The radiology department, in lots of cases, would not be able to complete their job if it weren't for the nurse's help. Refusing to help is not an option for the nurse. The system is set up so that we have to do it. We could get in trouble for not helping.

Now regardless of how busy the nurse is, if the nurse were to ask the radiology tech to perform a simple function, such as emptying a Foley catheter, the radiology tech would face no complications for refusing to do it. Emptying a Foley catheter can be performed by a non-licensed person. But again, since the radiologist cannot do the X-ray alone in some cases, such as the patient being too heavy or not cooperating, again, the nurse must help. The nurse cannot refuse to help because the X-ray must get done. There are lots of times, after the orders are put in for the X-rays, that the nurse must call the X-ray department because they never showed up to take the X-ray. The orders for the x-ray goes directly to the X-ray department. When this happens, this is more time taken away from nursing duties. The nurse now is alerting the X-ray department that they have X-rays to do. This is a call that should not have had to be made by the nurse. Again, the radiology department receives the X-ray orders. These delays in the X-ray tech showing up lots of times delays the patient from being transferred or discharged, further slowing down the nurse's job. It also has made patients upset, and the patient's anger is usually directed at the nurse, who is the only one that the patient sees on a continual basis. The patient does not always realize that this is out of the nurse's control.

There are times when the X-ray is not taken properly. In some of these cases, it may delay a patient from being transferred or possibly going home until the X-ray tech shows up and performs the X-ray again. This, too, will slow the nurses down, especially if the nurse has to help the X-ray tech so that he can perform the X-ray. If the X-ray tech is late showing up and the doctor is waiting to see the X-ray, the doctor will almost always call the nurses to ask them what the holdup is. This is after the doctor knows that the X-ray department has received the X-ray order. This now forces the nurse to call the X-ray department when the doctor himself should have called the X-ray department to find out why there is a holdup.

There are those times when a patient needs an X-ray and they will need things removed from them, like a brace or a partial cast or the like, so that the X-ray can be effectively taken. In this case, the radiologist usually needs the nurse's help in removing these objects. Once the X-ray is taken, the nurse usually puts these objects back where they belong on the patient. Here, again, is a case of the radiologist needing the nurse to complete his job. When X-rays are not taken properly by the radiologist, the X-ray has to be retaken. There have been many times to count, when the radiologist has reawakened or caused pain for a patient whom the nurse just managed to keep quiet from the earlier X-ray. This is no problem for the radiologist. He only has to retake the X-ray. The problem now falls on the nurse who has to work on keeping the patient quiet and comfortable all over again. The patient, if upset, is upset with the nurse, not realizing that it was the radiologist's mistake.

Nurses and patients are sometimes delayed because of X-ray reports that are not complete. For example, when a patient has a port or an opti-flow catheter inserted, which is a device that allows a patient to have dialysis, the insertion of these devices can sometimes cause the patient to develop a pneumothorax, which is a hole in the lung. The radiology report should specifically state if there is a pneumothorax or not, and when the report does not state this, it is the nurse that calls the radiology department, pointing out what is missing on the report. Here, the nurse is helping the radiology department with their job.

Lots of times, the X-ray tech needs a patient's extremity positioned with a blanket or towel. It is the nurse that must stop what she is doing to give the X-ray tech that towel or blanket. The X-ray tech realizes that sometimes they may need those supplies, but they never think to bring them. At times, the radiologist, not being too sure of an X-ray order, will ask the nurse if he or she is sure that this is what the doctor wants, when the nurses have no idea what the doctor wants, since it was the doctor who put the order in. Sometimes the X-ray department will call the nurse and tell the nurse the results of an X-ray. This call to the nurse should never happen. The nurse can do nothing about the patient's X-ray results. This is a call that should have gone to the doctor who ordered the X-ray. Nurses, however, continue to take these things. Nurses can sometimes be nuts for allowing these things to happen.

The radiologist's job is important to patient care, but if the nurse does not help the radiologist when he needs help, the nurse will get into trouble. Lots of times, when the radiologist comes to take an X-ray, it is the nurse who tells the radiologist which patient to take the X-ray on.

Sometimes doctors put what is called a central line in the patient. After the central lines are put in the patient, an X-ray is required to make sure that the central line is in the right place. If the central line is not in the right place, the radiology department will always call the nurse to tell her that the central line is not in the correct place. This is a call that should go to the doctor who put the central line in and not the nurse.

When the X-ray tech takes an X-ray on a patient, he must do something to the X-ray machine so that the radiologist can read the X-rays. When this is not done to the machine, sometimes the X-ray department will tell the nurse to tell the X-ray tech to fix the machine so that the radiologist can read the X-ray. The X-ray department should tell the X-ray tech to do this. This is not the nurse's job. All X-ray reports must be documented by the radiologist. Sometimes this is not done. This is particularly troubling for a patient who needs his X-ray report before going home. When this documentation is not done in a timely manner by the radiologist, the nurse must call radiology and tell them to document the report.

Sometimes patients will get upset with the nurse for not being discharged in a timely manner, not realizing that this is not the nurse's fault. Nurses do not get paid extra to be a radiologist. Nurses are nuts for letting these things happen.

LABORATORY DEPARTMENT

There are times when blood samples need to be drawn on patients for different reasons, such as for a complete blood-count test (CBC), a basic metabolic panel (BMP), and other tests. These tests are usually drawn by a phlebotomist, who is a person who draws blood tests. There are instances when the phlebotomists do not show up. There are also times when the phlebotomists are unable to draw blood samples for various reasons, for instance, because of an uncooperative patient or because of a patient who has bad veins. In either case, the blood has to be drawn, and when the phlebotomist cannot do it, the nurse must do it. What we have here is the nurse doing the phlebotomist's job. The nurse is not compensated anything extra for being the phlebotomist. The job must be done, and if it is not done, the blame will fall on the nurse.

There are times when the nurse has to call the lab department after the lab order has been put in to see when the phlebotomist will be coming to draw the labs. When orders for labs go on the computer, the lab department receives the order. This is a call the nurse should not have to make but often does. The lab also has a habit of asking the nurse what the patient's name is who needs labs drawn. This is a question that does not need to be asked since the person answering the phone is not coming to draw the labs.

There are times when, for whatever reason, the patient's upper extremities cannot be used for lab draws. In this case, the patient's lower extremities must be used instead. The phlebotomist, in most cases, is not allowed to draw blood from a patient's lower extremities.

When this is the case, it is the nurse who is left to do the job. In my opinion, the phlebotomist should have the authorization to use a patient's lower extremity for blood draws.

There are times when a patient's transfer is delayed because the phlebotomist does not show up in a timely manner, which is not good if the patient is, for example, in a recovery room and has to move out to make room for new patients that have to go to the recovery room. When this happens, it is usually the nurse that gets blamed for the patient not moving. If the nurse can, he will try to draw the labs himself to speed up the process, and here again, the nurse is doing the phlebotomist's job.

After the labs are drawn, the nurses usually wait until the results are back, and sometimes, it takes a while for the results to come back because the lab department has lots of patients they are working on. There are other times when the labs are lost or they did not get to the correct department in the lab to be resulted and the nurse must call the lab department. When this is the case, if it were not for the nurse calling the lab department, there is a good chance that the lab may not be resulted. When this happens, it is the nurse's call that has alerted the lab department that the lab must be found and resulted. This happens quite often, and here again, the nurse is involved with helping the lab complete their job.

Sometimes labs are timed. This means that labs are ordered to be drawn at a certain time. Now in all fairness to the lab, sometimes they show up, and the patient is not there. Other times, the lab does not get there on time to draw them. When the results are not back when the doctor is looking for them, he immediately confronts the nurses to ask them what the delay is. It seems to never occur to him to call the lab and ask them if they have drawn the labs yet. The lab department did receive the doctor's order, yet again, the nurse must call the lab department to get the ball rolling.

You have times when a patient is not stable and stat labs are required. The lab department does not always show up in time, yet the patient is unstable and needs labs drawn right away. When this happens, it is the nurse who must draw the labs. If these labs are not immediately drawn and the patient's condition continues to deteriorate, it is the nurses who will get blamed and not the lab department. In lots of cases, when the phlebotomist comes to draw the patient's blood, they do not know which patient to go to. This happens quite a bit in the post-anesthesia care unit. What the phlebotomist should do is check the patient's identification bracelet. They usually will ask the nurse to identify the patient instead. Here we have a situation where the nurse is taking time out of his day to do what the phlebotomist is capable of doing on his own. Lots of times, the phlebotomist will ask a sleeping patient his name and age. When the patient does not answer, the phlebotomist will ask the nurse this same information. The patient wears an identification bracelet, so in this case, the phlebotomist is supposed to look at the patient's identification bracelet. It is the same thing the nurse has to do!

Lots of times, when labs are drawn, there is certain equipment that has to come off of the patient, like a BP cuff. There are numerous times when the phlebotomist will not put this equipment back on and, in lots of cases, fail to tell the nurse that the equipment was removed. In some cases, the phlebotomist will not draw the patient's labs because he said he does not have an order even though the order is there and it is shown to the phlebotomist by the nurse. If the phlebotomist did not get the order, it was because he was on another lab run. When the phlebotomist does not draw the labs and the results are not back, the doctor gets mad at the nurse.

The phlebotomists have very busy jobs. They are called on for blood draws all over the hospital. Sometimes they can be short-staffed, and that is a problem, making it hard for them to be prompt. If this is the case, the phlebotomists will not get in any trouble for not showing up. If the patient experiences any problems or even if the patient dies, the phlebotomist will more than likely not get in trouble. It is a great position to be in, knowing that if you did not do your job, you would face no consequences. The phlebotomists are always in a position wherein if they don't show up in a timely manner, even if staffing is no problem, they will not face the consequences.

Lots of times, when labs are drawn, the lab department will need what is known as a confirmation. A lot of times, the lab department will tell the nurse to tell that person drawing the blood this instead of telling them themselves. The nurse often wastes a lot of time on the phone with the lab department. Sometimes before the phlebotomists come to draw the labs that are needed, the lab department will call the nurse to ask for the patient's name. This is a call that the nurses should not have to answer because the lab department has the patient's name in the order.

Sometimes patients have lines that the nurse can draw blood from, thereby not needing a phlebotomist. These are lines that look like the lines that you can draw blood from, but you cannot draw blood from these lines. Sometimes when the phlebotomist shows up, they will tell that nurse she could have drawn the blood herself from the line. The nurse has to explain to the phlebotomist that blood cannot be drawn from that particular line. Because the phlebotomist knows nothing about lines, this is a particular conversation that should never take place.

Sometimes, before the patient goes into the operating room, they will need a type and cross done. This is a test to determine a patient's blood type. Sometimes extra tubes are needed to complete this test. If extra tubes were needed to complete the test and they were not drawn, the test cannot be completed. Sometimes, when the patient makes it to the operating room and needs blood and cannot get it because the extra tubes were not drawn, the operating room nurse will sometimes call the nurse in the preoperative area and tell her that the extra tubes were not drawn. This call should have gone to the lab since there is nothing the preoperative nurse can do about it.

There are times when labs are due, usually at night, when the lab department has to be called to draw labs. Sometimes they do not answer the phone, and when this happens, the nurse has to walk to the lab department. Nurses do not get paid extra to be a phlebotomist. Nurses are nuts for letting these things happen.

PHYSICAL THERAPY DEPARTMENT

Physical therapists help injured or ill people improve their movement and manage their pain. Physical therapists can be found lots of times on the patients' floors, working with them.

There are times when the physical therapist can have a difficult patient, be it mentally or physically. The nurse is routinely asked to assist by giving meds, helping the physical therapist get the patent out of bed to the chair, or by helping the physical therapist walk with the patient.

Physical therapy is a part of the patient's care, and it must be done. The problem is, nurses on the floors have numerous patients that they are taking care of at one time, and when they have to help the physical therapist, it takes them from other things that they are doing. These situations arise from time to time with the physical therapists and patients, and the nurse is expected to help the physical therapist. There are times when the patients are being discharged when they have to be taught things such as crutch training. In lots of cases, this is the physical therapist's job to do, but it is something that routinely falls on the nurse's shoulders.

In lots of cases, the physical therapist may be done for the day and have gone home for the day. In that case, the nurse must do the physical therapist's job (the nurse is not compensated anything extra for being the physical therapist). The physical therapist will still be compensated for a full day's work that the nurses have helped him with. When the physical therapist is not around, nurses can be found helping patients with their range of motion exercises twenty-four-seven. The physical therapist does this eight hours a day. Again, the nurses are working with the patients twenty-four hours a day.

Patients need crutches, walkers, and overhead trapeze set up on beds. These pieces of equipment need to be set up. It is what the physical therapist should do, but the nurse, from time to time, will set these things up herself. When the nurses do this, it saves the physical therapist from doing it, so again, the nurse has done the physical therapist's job.

Patients who have had knee procedures are sometimes placed in continuous passive motion (CPM) machines, which exercise the knee. The physical therapists set this up, but nurses have been known to also set up these machines for patients. The physical therapist will sometimes go to the nurse to get information that can be found in the patient's chart. If the patient went home and had a problem, say with crutches, that physical therapist should have taught them but did not, then the nurse has to do it. The nurse could get into trouble even though the nurse did what physical therapy failed to do.

There are times when the physical therapist will need to point out a new finding with the patient to the doctor. Sometimes, the physical therapist will tell the nurse to tell the doctor about the finding instead of telling the doctor herself.

The nurse, lots of times, will talk to the physical therapist about the patient's activity level and diet level. These are things the physical therapist can do on his own by reading the patient's chart and by talking to the patient. When patients need crutch and walker training before they go home, they can only do it with a doctor's order. There are lots of times when the doctor forgets to put this order in. In lots of cases, the physical therapist will tell the nurse to let the doctor know that this order is needed. The physical therapist who needs this order should be the one notifying the doctor, not the nurse. Nurses do not get paid extra to be a physical therapist. Nurses are nuts for letting these things happen.

HEALTH-UNIT
COORDINATORS (HUCS)

All hospitals have HUCs who are health-unit coordinators. They are responsible for things like assembling charts, answering phones, and entering patient information into the computer. Now, when these functions cannot be performed, it is the nurse who usually picks up the slack.

Sometimes the HUCs get very busy, and the nurse will usually help out in these instances. There are times when the HUC may be sick or on vacation. When this is the case, a lot of the time, the nurses will be required to do the HUC's job. When nurses are sick, no one can do our duty except for another nurse, which usually leads to the nurses being short-staffed. Again, we have a situation where the nurse is expected to do someone else's job. If the nurse does not do it, it will not get done, and the HUC's job must be done in order for the units to function effectively. If it does not get done, the nurses will get blamed. The nurse is not compensated anything extra in this case for being the HUC. When the HUC takes a lunch or dinner break, the nurse must do the HUC's job. When the nurse takes a lunch or dinner break, the HUC cannot do the nurse's job. When the HUC is on vacation, the nurse must do the HUC's job. When the nurse is on vacation, the HUC cannot do the nurse's job.

Covering for the HUC's is something that nurses do a lot, and they get no extra appreciation for it, but the nurses allow this to happen. Nurses complain about these situations from time to time but never come together to force some changes, so the above continues. The nurse should not have to do the HUC's job. There should always be an HUC on duty. There should always be an HUC to cover another HUC while he is on break or vacation. Nurses are nuts for not demanding changes here. Sad to say though, the predicament that the nurse finds himself in is expected. The HUCs expect the nurses to step in and cover their duties when they're busy and are not there, and sadly enough, too many nurses themselves feel that they must do these duties. The HUC will still be compensated for a full day's work that the nurse helped her with.

The HUCs are also responsible for consulting other doctors on patients. These calls can be time-consuming. Nurses sometimes get stuck doing these consults when they should be taking care of their patients. Sometimes, on these consult calls, insurance problems arise, further using up the nurse's time.

There are times when the doctor consulted does not have privileges at the hospital. Now the nurse must call the doctor who asked for the consult to find out what other doctor he wants. The nurse should not have to do this, but she does it over and over again. There are times when new patients arrive on units, and they have charts that must be put together, which is the HUC's job. The nurse can be found doing this job also.

The phone can be and usually is answered by anyone. There are, however, lots of times when the phone is ringing and the HUC can be tied up for whatever reason and the nurse has to answer the phone even though the nurse may also be tied up with patient care.

HUCs are responsible for entering information into the computers such as when a patient is transferred from one place to another. Nurses have been known to perform this function if the HUC is off for the day or cannot get around to it for whatever reason. In certain areas, the doctors will enter the nurse's needed orders on the computer. It is the HUC's job to print up these orders for the nurse. Sometimes the HUC is not around, and sometimes the HUC forgets to do it. In any of these cases, it is the nurse who must print up the orders. I cannot tell you how many times the HUCs get upset with the nurses when the nurses do not hear what they said at first, not realizing that the nurses are extremely busy taking care of patients.

Sometimes when patients are brought to the floor, the HUC will tell the nurse that the patient's registration cannot be found. This is not the nurse's fault or responsibility, and the HUC knows this. The HUC knows that in a situation like this, the registration office is to be called.

When nurses bring patients to the floor, the nurse will sometimes keep the patient's chart in order to give the receiving nurse that patient's report. Sometimes the patient's chart will be left in the room. When the chart is left in the room, it is the HUC's job to go and get the chart. Lots of times, the HUC will tell the nurse to go and get the patient's chart. This is not the nurse's job. Nurses are nuts for allowing these things to happen.

I am not saying that the HUC's job is not important. His job is vital. What I am saying is that if he does not do his job, it usually falls on the nurse, and if it does not get done, it is the nurse who will get blamed.

Sometimes the phone can be ringing, and the HUC could be on the phone, and the nurse could be busy, and another nurse will yell out to that nurse to answer the phone instead of telling the HUC to put her call on hold and to answer the phone.

When patients are transferred to another floor, they must be transferred into the receiving floor's computer, and the HUC is supposed to do the transfer. Sometimes the HUC will tell the nurse to make the transfer. The nurse is not trained to do this, nor is it the nurse's job. Nurses do not get paid extra to be an HUC. Nurses are nuts for letting these things happen.

PHARMACY DEPARTMENT

The pharmacy department plays a vital role in hospitals. They prepare and dispense medications. Sometimes the pharmacist will receive an order from the doctor on a med whose written dosage he is not sure of. In some cases, the pharmacist will call the nurse in order to get clarification on this. The problem here is that the nurse did not write the order. The nurse does not have authorization to write the order. The appropriate thing for the pharmacist to do is to call the doctor on this. We, in turn, tell the pharmacist to call the doctor. The pharmacist knows that this should have been done in the first place. The problem here is that the nurse has wasted valuable time talking to the pharmacist about something he should have never been called on, but this situation happens frequently. Here, we have a situation where the pharmacist is hoping that the nurse can do the doctor's job.

There are cases when the nurse tells the pharmacist what he thinks the doctor's order may be, and if the pharmacist thinks it makes sense, he will go with what the nurse suggested. In this situation, the nurse has helped the doctor also. The doctor has been helped because this saves him a call from the pharmacist. When the pharmacist calls the nurse, it does not matter how busy the nurse is; the nurse must talk to the pharmacist. If the pharmacist is in the nurse's presence and the nurse asks the pharmacist to get him extra linen, the pharmacist will not get into trouble for refusing to help. The pharmacist will sometimes ask the nurse to check with the doctor to get a clarification on a particular medication order that the pharmacist thinks is wrong. The pharmacist should have to question the medical order. Sometimes the nurse will call the doctor to get clarification that is needed, which saves the pharmacist from doing his job. Things like this happen over and over again, and nurses are nuts for allowing it to keep happening.

There are times when the nurses are out of a certain medication, and when this happens, the pharmacy is the one who should come to restock the medication. This does not always happen, but sometimes the pharmacy will send the medication to the nurse's station, making the nurse restock the med. This should not happen! The nurse may not be able to get the med in a timely manner to stock it. The med could be taken by someone, and if that happens, the nurse would probably get blamed. The pharmacy is responsible for stocking narcotics. In most cases, the nurse is not there to verify the count of the narcotic being stocked by the pharmacy. If the pharmacist makes a counting mistake, which has happened before, the nurse bears the blame when she goes to remove the narcotic if the count is off. The nurse should always be involved with the pharmacist to verify the count when the narcotic is being stocked.

Medications that have been given and medication orders are routinely set up to the pharmacist. Sometimes the penmanship on these orders is not clear. It is not uncommon for the pharmacist to call the nurse to ask her if she can understand the medication order that the doctor has written. The nurse will always try to help the pharmacist understand the order. The problem here is that the nurse may interpret the reading wrong or may not understand the written order herself. What the pharmacist should do in cases like these is call the doctor himself to get clarification on the order.

When the pharmacy department fills the Pyxis machine, a nurse should always be with the person filling the Pyxis to make sure that the medication count is correct, but this is not always the case. A Pyxis is an automated medication-dispensing system. Nurses are nuts for letting this happen.

The pharmacist is very important, and his job is vital, but if the nurse does not help the pharmacist, the nurse will get in trouble. There are medications that should be dosed by a pharmacist to give to patients. The pharmacist does not always do this. When it is not done, the nurse has to do it since the patient must get the ordered medication. Medications are held in a machine called a Pyxis. The pharmacy department puts these medications in the Pyxis. There are a lot of times when the medication the nurse goes for is not in the Pyxis. In this case, the nurse has to call the pharmacy so that they can put the medication in the Pyxis or leave their department and go to a Pyxis in another department. At times, the nurse may badly need the medication. This should never happen. The pharmacy should always make sure that the Pyxis is filled. If the patient takes a turn for the worse because he did not get the medication on time, it is the nurse and not the pharmacy who will get in trouble.

There are times when the pharmacy is supposed to be monitoring an intravenous medication that the patient is getting. An intravenous medication is one that is set up on a pump and goes through the patient's vein. A lot of times, the pharmacist will call the nurse and ask the nurse what the pump is set at instead of coming to check the pump himself.

There have been times when a patient has left the hospital to get a prescription filled at a pharmacy and the pharmacist is not too sure what quantity to fill the prescription. The outside pharmacy usually calls the nurse to get clarification on the prescription when it is the hospital pharmacy that should be called about this matter. The nurse should not be called about this.

There are times when the pharmacy department is filling the Pyxis machine (a machine that dispenses medication) and the nurse must get in there to give an emergent medication to a patient. When this happens, the pharmacy department sometimes will not stop filling the Pyxis machine to allow the nurse to get her medication in a timely manner. This is unacceptable behavior on the part of the pharmacy department because the nurse's medication administration is very important, and some of the medications that the pharmacy fills the Pyxis with, the nurse does anyway. Nurses do not get paid extra for being a pharmacist. Nurses are nuts for letting these things happen.

RESPIRATORY THERAPY DEPARTMENT

Respiratory therapists care for patients who have trouble breathing. They administer breathing treatments, draw arterial blood gas samples on people, and perform other various functions.

There are patients in the hospital, at various times, that run into problems breathing. When this happens, the patient may need a respiratory treatment, ventilator support, or both. The job of the respiratory therapist is to provide that support.

Sometimes, the respiratory therapist is tied up and cannot come to the patient who needs help right away. If the patient cannot get help quickly, that patient will suffer. In these cases, nurses have been known to give the patient the respiratory care that is needed, which can include mask treatments or setting up a ventilator for a patient if needed. If the respiratory therapist does not show up in a timely manner and the nurse does not step in, the patient could die. The nurse is not compensated anything extra, in this case, for being the respiratory therapist. The respiratory therapist is an important part of the healthcare team and performs a vital role in the patient's care, but if he is busy and does not show up in a timely manner or if the department is short-staffed, which results in a bad outcome for the patient, it will be the nurse who is ultimately liable. The respiratory therapist who has been notified to show up stat can use the excuse that he was busy or short-staffed for not showing up right away. Regardless of how busy the nurse is with other patients, if one of his patients has a respiratory emergency that ends up bad for the patient, that nurse cannot use the "I was too busy with another patient" excuse. Yet the nurse could be so busy that he might have to ask the respiratory therapist for a urinal or bed pan, and if the respiratory therapist refuses, he faces no consequences. The nurse does the respiratory therapist's job routinely, and there is no thanks in return for doing it, and this is a problem.

The respiratory therapist should be held to a higher standard. They may say that they are short staffed, but, no one is more short-staffed than the nursing department, yet the nurse still finds a way to do the respiratory therapist's job. Nurses should demand change. Nurses should demand that respiratory therapists are always there to do their job. Nurses should let it be known that they routinely do the respiratory therapist's job. Nurses should let it be known that it impacts their care for other patients while they are doing the respiratory therapist's job. Nurses are nuts for not fighting to change these things. Nurses are short-staffed regularly, but they still get their job done and the job of others. The respiratory therapist should not be able to use excuses such as being too busy, short-staffed, or not arriving in a timely manner, but he uses these excuses and gets away with it. To repeat, if a patient with a respiratory emergency has a bad outcome due to the respiratory therapist not arriving in a timely manner, the nurse will bear the blame, and that is not right.

Now I understand that the patient is under the nurse's care. The patient in the OR is under the surgeon's care, but surgery would not be successful without everyone doing their part. For example, the anesthesiologists, the OR techs, and the nurses all play a hand in helping the surgeon. The funny thing here is that the nurse often gets the job done without help from the respiratory therapist. This respiratory therapist will still be compensated for a full day's work that the nurse helped him with. It is not unusual to have a patient on a ventilator that is on a mechanical ventilator and needs ventilator-setting changes. The respiratory therapist is called for this. Sometimes it takes the respiratory therapist a while to show up, in the meantime, these ventilator settings sometimes need to be made ASAP. For the patient's safety, it is not uncommon for the nurse to make the ventilator changes himself. A lot of times, when it is known that a patient will need a mechanical ventilator, the respiratory therapist will bring the ventilator to where it is needed. Now the respiratory therapist is the one who should place the patient on the ventilator, but if the patient has not shown up (e.g., a patient coming out of the operating room), sometimes the respiratory therapist will leave, leaving the nurse with the responsibility of placing the patient on the ventilator. In this case, the nurse has done the respiratory therapist's job.

Arterial blood gases are sometimes needed on patients. Arterial blood gases are tests that measure the levels of oxygen and carbon dioxide in the blood. The blood is obtained by drawing blood from the radial artery via a needle stick or drawing the blood from an arterial line that is already in the radial artery. This is a job for the respiratory therapist, but nurses routinely do this. Nurses will do chest percussion on a patient. Chest percussion is done on patients to help loosen and remove mucous from the lungs. It is a respiratory therapist's job, but nurses also do it on patients. Nurses do not get paid extra to be a respiratory therapist. Nurses are nuts for letting these things happen.

HOUSEKEEPING
DEPARTMENT

Hospital housekeepers are responsible for sustaining a sterile environment in all areas of the hospital by cleaning rooms, making beds, replenishing linens, and maintaining floors.

What usually happens in a hospital is that, when a patient is transferred or discharged, housekeeping is notified so that the room can be cleaned in order to receive a new patient. There are times when housekeepers have so many rooms to clean that it causes a delay for patients that need to go to the room. In these instances, it is not uncommon for a nurse to clean rooms in order to speed up placing patients in rooms. The nurse is not compensated anything extra in this case for being the housekeeper. However, in order to keep the patient flow moving as best as possible, we do it. Now, this is a chore that can take a nurse away from his patients for some time, but in some cases, the nurse must do it.

If the housekeeper is cleaning a bed and the nurse is caring for a patient in the neighboring bed and that patient becomes nauseous and the nurse asks the housekeeper for an emesis basin, and the housekeeper refuses to get it, the housekeeper will not get in trouble. I am not saying that the housekeeper would not get the emesis basin because they probably would. I am just pointing out that if she does not do it, she faces no consequences, and it has no impact on the housekeeper's job. On the other hand, if the nurse does not help out with the housekeeping duties, it will have an effect on the nurse's job.

It is not uncommon for a housekeeper to remove a bed from a room when the room is being cleaned. Sometimes the housekeeper will not put the bed back in the room. When this happens, it is the nurse who puts the bed back into the room. There are times when the housekeeper is in the room, cleaning the beds, and the nurse will go to the housekeeper and tell her that she needs a specific bed cleaned first because a patient is waiting for that specific bed. Sometimes, the housekeeper, for whatever reason, will not clean the bed first that the nurse asked for, further causing a delay for the patient's arrival to the room. When the housekeeper is done cleaning a bed, she is supposed to enter into the computer that the bed is clean. Now it usually takes no more than thirty minutes to clean a bed, yet sometimes, much more than thirty minutes has passed by, and still, nothing is on the computer. In this case, the nurse usually goes to see if the bed is cleaned, and most of the time, it is. This move puts further work on the nurse and delays the patient from moving.

There are times when special occasions come up and people are visiting the hospital right where the head nurses want the area clean for. Sometimes the head nurses will ask the nursing staff to come in and help clean the hospital. This should not be. Housekeepers are the ones who should be doing this cleaning. Nurses do not get paid extra to be a housekeeper. Nurses are nuts for allowing these things to happen.

ORDERLIES / TRANSPORTERS

Orderlies are non-licensed hospital assistants. They are also called transporters. They can do a variety of things, such as transporting patients, making beds, bathing patients, recording intakes and outputs, and other things. When the orderly is there for the RN to help transport or to record an intake and output (I&O), it makes the nurse's job easier.

There are many occasions when the nurse is left to do this on his own. Performing an I&O, while sometimes time consuming, is not too bad. The big problem is when the nurse is required to bathe a patient without help and when she is expected to transport the patient. It is not uncommon to have a heavy patient, weight-wise, that a smaller nurse is forced to bathe and transport on her own. The transporting part really becomes tricky because the nurses have and can become injured, but, if the orderly is not around, the job still has to get done. If the job does not get done, the nurse is left to answer.

There are lots of times when the patient needs to be transferred or needs to go to X-ray or some other place in the hospital. There are times when the patient is discharged and has to be taken to their car, but if the orderlies or the transport person is not there, the nurse has to do it. Most times, the nurse has other patients that she is taking care of, but when a patient has to be moved, it is the nurse who has to do it if no one else is around. When the orderlies/transport team starts, while their job can be demanding, this is the only job that they have to concentrate on for the day.

If the nurse has a Foley catheter that needs emptying and the orderly cannot get around to it at the end of the day, he suffers no consequences for not doing it. If the nurse does not complete the orderly's job, for example, transferring a patient or taking a patient to a test, it is the nurse who gets blamed. This happens over and over again, and the nurse accepts it. Now sometimes the orderlies can be working with a limited staff and cannot always be there exactly when the nurse calls, but if that particular patient's care is not carried out, the orderly suffers no consequences even though it is his job to transfer the patient, take a patient to a test, or help the nurse with patient transferring. If the orderly cannot carry out his duty, the nurse must do it. The nurse is not compensated anything extra for being the orderly.

When patients come out of the operating room, patients are preferably put on beds instead of stretchers to avoid the patient having to move twice. If a bed has to be picked up, this is usually the orderly's job, yet nurses can be found countless times picking up the beds themselves. This should not happen, yet the nurse continually allows it. Going to pick up a bed takes time and energy. It takes the nurse away from his patients, and it exacts an extra physical toll on the nurse.

There are times when the orderly may be off for the day. In this case, the transporting duties will fall squarely on the nurse. There is no guarantee that the nurse will get help from anyone. Nurses then are forced, yet again, to do the orderly's job. Nurses allow this to happen over and over again. Things like this have been going on for so long because it is the way the system is set up. The nurse, if they wanted to be heard, would have a tough time finding someone to hear their complaints. Nurses could probably cover more ground in this area if they came together to let it be known that they routinely do the orderly's job. The sad thing about the situation is that the nurse routinely accepts this on top of the duties that he already has. The orderlies cannot help the nurses with their jobs, like giving medications, inserting NG tubes, and extensive dressing changes, just to name a few. The nurse must do her job and at times, she must do the orderly's job and this is not right. The orderly will still be compensated for a full day's work that the nurse helped him with.

There are times when the orderly will come to the floor to pick up a patient for a test. When this happens, the patient is usually taken off of his bed and placed on a transport stretcher. Sometimes the orderly or transporter is unable to do this on his own. When he is unable to do this, he gets the nurse to help him. Regardless of how busy the nurse may be with other duties, she will help the transporter out.

When patients go into the operating room, their beds are supposed to be outside of the operating room, waiting for the patient. It is supposed to be the orderly's job to get these beds. Sometimes they do not get the bed, which leaves this duty to fall on the nurse. Patients that are going to the operating room for certain procedures sometimes need a shave and a prep. This consists of cleaning hair away from the area that the surgery is going to be performed on. The orderlies are supposed to do this, but sometimes, they don't for various reasons. When the orderlies do not do it, it falls on the nurse to do it. It must be done, and if the job is not done, the nurse will get into trouble.

There are times when a patient is sleeping when the orderlies will wake that patient up to ask the patient if he is okay. Chances are that the sleeping patient is okay. If the patient cannot go back to sleep, it is the nurse that is stuck with this problem. If the patient takes a sleeping pill to fall asleep, he cannot be given another one. If the patient now needs a sleeping pill to go back to sleep, the nurse has to call the doctor to get an order for a sleeping pill, and if it is too late, the patient cannot be given a sleeping pill. The nurse now is stuck with trying to rectify a problem that should have never been.

In the preoperative area, the patients that have to go to the operating room (OR) are on stretchers. When the patients are ready to go to the OR, an OR nurse is supposed to be accompanied by an orderly. Sometimes the OR nurse cannot get an orderly to help her. When this happens, the nurse must push the stretcher herself or get a nurse that may be busy to help her bring the patient to the room.

This should not happen, but if the patient does not get to the OR room in time, it will be blamed on the nurse.

When an orderly takes a break, there should always be at least one available to help out the nurse if needed. However, it is not uncommon for a lot of the orderlies to all be on break at the same time. When JCAHO (Joint Commission on Accreditation of Health Care Organization) comes around, they will check the hallways a lot of times to make sure that stretchers and beds are not there, which can become a hazard in the case of a fire. Sometimes the orderlies will not put the stretchers and beds where they belong and will leave them in the hallways. If they are left in the hallways and the nurse knows that JCAHO is coming, the nurse is the one who ends up putting the stretchers where they belong because JCAHO could cite them for this, and it is the nurses who will get into trouble and not the orderlies.

When patients are discharged from the hospital, they must go by wheelchairs. Wheelchairs are usually stored in specific areas by the transporters and orderlies. There are times, late in the evening, when the transporters and orderlies are not around to help discharge a patient. In this case, the nurse must discharge the patient. There have been numerous times when the nurse cannot find a wheelchair because the transporters and orderlies did not put the wheelchair back where it belonged. In this case, the nurse is left to run around to look for a wheelchair so that the patient can be discharged. This is time consuming and something that the nurse should not have to do.

When in-house patients have to go for surgery, it is the transporter's and orderly's job to go to the patient's room to pick the patient up and bring the patient to pre-op. For whatever reason, the transporters and orderlies do not always do this, and when it is not done, the nurses have to do it. When the nurses do this, it takes away from the time they have to get the patient ready for surgery. This could also cause the patient to be late for surgery. If the patient is late for surgery, the doctors will blame the nurse and not the transporters and orderlies when they were the ones who failed to pick up the patient in the first place.

When patients are discharged from the hospital, in the recovery room, the stretcher must be moved from that spot since more patients will be coming. It is the orderly's and transporter's job to move these stretchers. Sometimes they do not move the stretchers, and when that happens, the nurse has to move the stretchers, and that puts extra work on the nurse.

There are times when the nurse needs the orderlies to do things, like taking a patient's blood-sugar level because the nurse is too busy at the time to do it herself. Taking a patient's blood-sugar level is an important function. Sometimes the orderly will tell the nurse that he is too busy making beds or moving stretchers, which is not an important function. When this happens, it forces the nurse to take on the added responsibility of taking the patient's blood-sugar level herself. Nurses do not get paid extra to be transporters and orderlies. Nurses are nuts for allowing these things to happen.

VOLUNTEER SERVICES IN HOSPITAL

Volunteers work in a variety of settings in the hospital. In the surgical area, they are a link between the operating room, recovery room, and the waiting room, with family members waiting for information on patients. Volunteers make the job of the nurse much easier when they relay information to family members about their loved ones. In the surgical setting, volunteers will let the family members know if their loved one is still in the operating room or recovery room.

Volunteers, however, are not always there. When their shifts end, they go home of course. In the surgical area, surgeries can go on around the clock. When the volunteers are not there, it is up to the nurse to take the role of a volunteer. It is now the nurse that must call or go to the waiting room and talk to the family member about what's going on with the patient. This takes time, and it often takes the nurse away from patient-care duties. Because the volunteers are not there twenty-four-seven, this becomes another job that the nurse undertakes.

Volunteers also answer the phones. Sometimes, for whatever reason, the volunteer will not answer the phone or is not there to answer it. In that case, it falls on the nurse to go to the waiting room to relay the information that the nurse is calling to tell the volunteer. This takes away from the nurse's time also. Nurses are nuts for allowing these things to happen. There are many times when the volunteers are told to bring a patient's family member to the perioperative area and the volunteers cannot find it. This forces the nurse to go get the family member. Nurses do not get paid extra to be a volunteer. Nurses are nuts for allowing these things to happen.

REGISTRATION DEPARTMENT

When patients get registered to the hospital, labels are created that are put on patient's charts and surgical consents. These labels sometimes have different account numbers than the numbers on the computer. When this happens, the nurse has to call registration to let them know that the labels have incorrect account numbers on them. There are times when the nurse tries to fix this problem herself, which is difficult because the nurse does not always have the proper equipment to make this change. In this case, the nurse must call registration to point out their mistake. If the patient is going into surgery, this can delay their surgery as it takes registration time to correct the problem and more time to send the correct labels to the waiting nurse.

Sometimes a discharged patient is readmitted to the hospital. There are times when the registration department has used the patient's discharge account number for the new admission. This causes all types of problems for the nurse, most notably, the ability to properly scan the patient's medication. When this happens, the nurse must call registration and tell them of their mistake, which takes time to clear up. In the meantime, the patient is forced to wait for the problem to be cleared up before they can get medicated or go to surgery.

When the patient is registered, they must be put down as a patient to be discharged or admitted to the hospital. Registration gets these orders from the doctor. Lots of times, registration puts these orders in the wrong, which makes it difficult for the patient to be either discharged or admitted. In either case, it is always the nurse who finds out this mistake and has to try to fix the problem or call registration to tell them to fix it.

Patients who have incorrect account numbers on their chart make it virtually impossible to charge for medications, and patients with the wrong labels with the incorrect account numbers on their chart can make the entire surgical process difficult because it can cause all types of billing problems if this number on the surgical consent is wrong. This can also cause a delay in charging the patients for surgery and the doctor getting his proper compensation for it. It is the nurse who always catches these incorrect labels.

There are also times when a discharged patient is readmitted to the hospital with his discharged account numbers on the labels. Again, if this happens, the patient cannot be given his proper medications because the labels do not match the account number on the computer. Again, it is always the nurse who discovers this and tries to fix it or contacts the registration department so that they can fix it. When these labels are wrong, it can delay a patient getting his proper care, which most of the time, involves his medications.

Also, when patients are registered for surgery, the registration department has orders from the doctor if the patient is going to be admitted or discharged. Sometimes registration does not record this properly and further slows the nurse down in either discharging the patient or getting an admission bed for the patient. Again, the nurse tries to fix this problem herself, but it sometimes is virtually impossible for the nurse to do this because she does not have the equipment for it. This delay usually upsets patients and their families tremendously. Sometimes the family members get upset with the nurse even though it is not the nurse's fault.

Nurses do not get paid extra to be registrars. Nurses are nuts for allowing these things to happen.

SECURITY DEPARTMENT

The security department in the hospital is designed to maintain safe grounds and to respond to the floor when the nurse calls concerning an unruly, dangerous, and threatening patient. When security arrives, they sometimes cannot control the patient themselves. When this happens, the nurse is left with possibly trying to give the patient medication to sedate him or calling the cops. The problem with calling the cops is if the patient is baker acted or not.

A baker act is something that provides individuals with emergency services and temporary detention for mental health evaluation and treatment when required, either on a voluntary or involuntary basis. When a patient is baker acted, he may not be able to be taken to jail. If the patient stays with the nurse and continues to be violent and if security cannot help, the nurse must now also become a security guard.

When the operating room nurses are on call ("on call" means to come to work for an emergency surgery case), they are supposed to let security know this so that security can get the information for that particular vehicle so they do not get a ticket. Security has been known to not record this information correctly and have given nurses tickets anyway. This makes the nurse have to physically go to security to let them know that they gave them the proper information so that the ticket can be taken away. This is very time consuming for the nurse.

Nurses do not get paid extra to be a security guard. Nurses are nuts for allowing these things to happen.

CONCLUSION

N urses have very hard jobs. In addition to what they do, they can be found helping other disciplines with their jobs or even doing other discipline's jobs entirely, from admitting patients to discharging them. It is the nurse who does this. Hospitals would not be able to function without the nurse being there. Again, the nurse helps everyone with their jobs, and there is no way that the nurse can avoid this because the system is set up where the nurse must always be there to help the other disciplines.

A doctor is capable of sitting down at a computer to look up labs on his patient, but a lot of the time, he will ask the nurse to do this for him, and the nurse cannot refuse.

X-rays are done a lot on patients in hospitals. It is always the nurse who tells the X-ray tech what patient to do the X-ray on. The X-ray tech who has the patient's name can easily identify the patient by looking at the patient's name band, but the X-ray tech will not do this most of the time. He finds it more convenient to ask a nurse to identify the patient for them.

Labs are drawn on patients routinely in hospitals by the phlebotomists. Since all patients have an ID bracelet, the phlebotomist has the name of the patient who needs the labs drawn. All the phlebotomist has to do is look at the patient's ID bracelet to see if he or she is the one who needs the labs. This is usually not done by the phlebotomist because the phlebotomist usually asks the nurse to identify the patient for him.

The physical therapist uses the nurse to help her out quite a bit. Nurses routinely inform the physical therapist about the patient's activity level and what the patient can or cannot eat.

The nurse helps the HUCs quite a bit as well and can be found printing up orders on patients, which is a job for the HUCs.

The nurse can be found helping the pharmacist quite a bit with tasks like clarifying a doctor's order and telling the pharmacist to call the doctor if clarification cannot be achieved.

The respiratory therapist is helped by the nurse often. There are times when the respiratory therapist does not make it in a timely fashion to give a patient a treatment that is needed. In this case, the nurse will sometimes administer the treatment herself.

Housekeepers are assigned with the duties of cleaning patients' rooms, but when they do not show up to clean in a timely fashion, which happens a lot, the nurse cleans the room.

Nurses routinely transport patients for transporters and orderlies. There are times when a patient must be transferred to a stretcher for transport, and sometimes the nurses can be found doing this job alone.

Volunteers, at times, update patient's families concerning the status of their loved one. They get this information from the nurse. When the volunteers aren't there, the nurse must do this herself.

There are many times when a patient is registered in the hospital, and his account numbers are wrong. When this happens, the nurse must try to correct this herself or call the registration department to correct it.

Sometimes security is called to go to the floor to help with unruly, dangerous patients. There are times when security cannot handle the patient they are called for. When this happens, the nurse must now become a security guard!

At the end of the day, nurses have a way of helping many hospital disciplines do their jobs while sometimes doing their job entirely. Nurses do all of this and receive no compensation. Nurses do not get paid to be the doctor, radiology tech, phlebotomist, physical therapist, HUC, pharmacist, respiratory therapist, housekeeper, transporter, volunteer, registration personnel, or security guard, yet they do their jobs willingly with no complaints. That's why I say nurses are nuts!

ABOUT THE AUTHOR

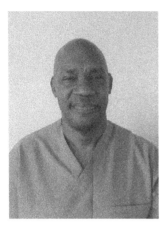

Anthony Langley has been a registered nurse for twenty-nine years now. He also has a bachelor's degree in criminal justice. He, at one time, wanted to become an attorney since attorneys were something his father talked about a lot.

His interest in nursing started after getting a job as a security officer in the emergency room of a hospital. There was a male nurse who worked in the emergency room who would show him lots of things that nurses did. This got him interested in nursing. He went to nursing school and got his bachelor's degree in nursing in 1990. At his first job, he started on a medical surgical unit, which is a unit that takes care of patients with different medical conditions and who have had surgery. From the medical surgical unit, he took a job in a surgical stepdown unit, where intensive care patients are transferred to when they stabilize. After this, he started on a surgical intensive care unit, which is where unstable surgical patients go to after surgery.

After about two years there, he began working on the same-day surgery unit, which is where people go to have surgery and are discharged home afterward. From the same-day surgery unit, he took a job in a post-anesthesia care unit (PACU) recovery room. Patients that go to the PACU unit are in-house patients who have had surgery. These surgeries can include orthopedic, gastric, and urological surgeries and more.

CPSIA information can be obtained
at www.ICGtesting.com
Printed in the USA
LVHW090324171219
640669LV00005B/906/P